Carnivore Diet for Women

A 14-Day Beginner's Step-by-Step Guide with Curated Recipes and a Meal Plan

mf

Disclaimer

This guide is intended solely for informational and educational purposes. It should not be interpreted as medical advice, diagnosis, or treatment. The author is not a physician, nurse, mental health provider, or registered dietitian, and reading this guide does not create any form of patient–provider relationship.

Always consult a licensed healthcare professional regarding any questions about your health, medical conditions, or before making changes to your diet, exercise, or lifestyle. Never delay, disregard, or substitute professional guidance based on information presented here.

The publisher and author disclaim responsibility for any adverse effects, outcomes, or consequences that may result from the use or application of the material in this guide. No specific results, benefits, or improvements are promised or guaranteed.

All product names, diet plans, and trademarks mentioned are the property of their respective owners and appear only for descriptive or identification purposes.

Table of Contents

Introduction — 5

What Is the Carnivore Diet? — 7

Who Should Not Follow the Carnivore Diet? — 16

The Benefits of the Carnivore Diet — 21

Potential Risks and Nutrient Gaps — 34

14-Day Guide to Stick to the Carnivore Diet Plan — 43

Easing into the Carnivore Diet — 49

Sample 14-Day Guide — 55

Sample 7-Day Carnivore Diet Meal Plan — 62

Long-Term Sustainability and Alternatives — 66

Sample Recipes — 74

Making the Change for Better Health — 97

Conclusion — 107

FAQs — 109

References and Helpful Links — 112

Introduction

Across wellness circles, more women are exploring the carnivore diet as a potential way to address stubborn health frustrations that often linger despite multiple attempts with other plans. Fatigue that doesn't lift with extra sleep, bloating that persists even with "healthy" foods, skin concerns that resist conventional fixes, or weight challenges that feel unshakable—these are some of the reasons women begin looking for alternative strategies. Hormonal shifts during the 30s, 40s, and beyond may add another layer of complexity, leading many to experiment with dietary approaches that promise simplicity and focus.

The carnivore diet is one such approach. Unlike keto or paleo, which allow at least some plant-based foods, carnivore is an elimination-style plan that centers entirely on animal foods.

This means meals are built around meat, fish, eggs, and sometimes dairy, while all fruits, vegetables, grains, legumes, nuts, and seeds are excluded. Excluding plants restricts the diet to animal foods only, a change that simplifies options but also limits nutrient diversity.

This guide was created to walk you through what the carnivore diet is, how it differs from other low-carb approaches, what the reported benefits and challenges are, and how some women structure their meals during the first few weeks. While many report improvements in energy, digestion, or mood, the diet remains highly restrictive and is not a universal solution. Nutritional adequacy, food variety within animal choices, and medical monitoring are essential considerations.

Most importantly, this guide is for educational purposes only. It is not medical advice and should not replace consultation with a qualified healthcare provider. Because the carnivore diet eliminates entire food groups, anyone considering it should first discuss the risks and suitability with a physician or registered dietitian.

What Is the Carnivore Diet?

The carnivore diet has drawn attention in recent years as one of the most restrictive approaches to eating. Unlike plans that allow for a range of food groups, this way of eating focuses exclusively on animal products. For some, its appeal lies in simplicity: there are no carb counts, portion charts, or complex meal rules. For others, it raises questions about balance, nutrients, and long-term sustainability.

To better understand the carnivore diet, it helps to compare it with the ketogenic (keto) diet, a more familiar low-carbohydrate plan. Both share features that can push the body into ketosis, but they differ in what foods are allowed, how they are tracked, and why people choose one approach over another.

Keto in Brief

The ketogenic diet has been used in various forms for decades. It is a high-fat, moderate-protein, very low-carbohydrate plan. By limiting carbohydrates to a narrow range—often around 20 to 50 grams per day—the body shifts from using glucose as its main fuel to producing ketones from fat.

Keto allows both animal and plant foods, as long as they fit within the carbohydrate limit. This can include:

- Meat, poultry, and fish
- Eggs and dairy (in moderation)
- Nuts, seeds, and low-carb vegetables such as leafy greens, zucchini, and cauliflower
- Healthy fats such as olive oil, butter, or avocado

Because the diet depends on keeping carbs consistently low, many people track macronutrients daily. This often involves weighing portions, checking nutrition labels, or using apps to stay in range.

Carnivore in Brief

The carnivore diet removes plant foods altogether. Meals are built only from animal products such as:

- Beef, pork, poultry, and lamb
- Fish and shellfish
- Eggs
- Some versions allow dairy, while stricter approaches focus on meat, salt, and water only

Supporters often describe carnivores as a "zero-carb" diet. There is no need to calculate macros because the food choices are so narrow. As long as meals stay within the animal kingdom, the rules are technically followed.

The narrow food list removes the need for tracking, but it also narrows the range of available nutrients. Plant-based fiber, antioxidants, and phytochemicals are absent, which is a central point of debate among health professionals.

Core Differences: Carnivore vs. Keto

When comparing carnivore to keto, the main differences come down to what foods are included and how much flexibility each approach allows. While both can shift the body toward ketosis, their rules and nutrient sources vary.

1. **Plant Inclusion**
   - *Keto*: Allows certain vegetables, nuts, seeds, and even low-sugar fruits in moderation.
   - *Carnivore*: Excludes all plant foods.

2. **Tracking**
   - *Keto*: Often requires tracking macronutrients to stay in ketosis.
   - *Carnivore*: No macro tracking—simplicity is part of the design.

3. **Flexibility**
   - *Keto*: Provides more food variety and recipe options.

- *Carnivore*: Extremely limited, which some find freeing and others find restrictive.

4. Nutrient Sources

- *Keto*: Fiber, vitamin C, magnesium, and plant compounds are still present.
- *Carnivore*: Relies on animal products for vitamins and minerals; some nutrients may be lower without careful planning.

These distinctions highlight why some people prefer the structure of carnivore while others find keto more sustainable. Understanding the trade-offs helps clarify which approach might align better with individual needs and goals.

Why Some Prefer Carnivore

The carnivore diet appeals to certain individuals because it removes much of the complexity that comes with other eating plans. Its straightforward rules can feel easier to follow, especially for those frustrated by food tracking or dietary restrictions.

1. Simplicity

For those tired of constant logging and tracking, the carnivore approach removes the extra steps and focuses only on eating.

2. **Plant Sensitivities**

Some individuals report digestive discomfort, bloating, or skin flare-ups from certain plant foods. Eliminating them can feel like a relief. While clinical research is limited, many women have noted subjective improvements, which contribute to the diet's growing interest.

3. **Rapid Structure**

People who want a clear "yes/no" framework sometimes find carnivores easier to follow than a diet that requires counting or portioning. The black-and-white rules reduce decision fatigue.

Although not suited to everyone, the simplicity and clarity of carnivore explain why it resonates with those seeking fewer choices and less dietary guesswork. These perceived benefits often outweigh its limitations for people drawn to its structure.

Why Others Do Better on Keto

For many people, keto provides a middle ground between carbohydrate restriction and dietary variety. By allowing both animal and select plant foods, it offers flexibility without abandoning the benefits of low-carb eating.

1. **Dietary Flexibility**

   Keto allows more variety, making it easier to enjoy social meals, cook creatively, and avoid boredom. The inclusion of vegetables also makes it easier to meet fiber and micronutrient needs.

2. **Long-Term Balance**

   Many find keto more sustainable because it doesn't cut out entire food groups. It may also be more adaptable to family meals or cultural cuisines.

3. **Nutrient Access**

   Keto eaters can benefit from the antioxidants and diverse nutrients that come from low-carb plant foods—something carnivores restrict.

This balance makes keto easier to maintain long term while supporting a wider range of nutrients. For those who value flexibility and sustainability, keto often proves to be the more practical choice.

Health Considerations

Both diets can lead to ketosis, which may support fat metabolism. But neither is automatically safe or appropriate for everyone. A few key points:

1. **Digestive Health**: Fiber from plants supports gut function. On carnivores, fiber intake drops to nearly zero, which may change bowel patterns. Some adapt; others struggle with constipation.

2. **Micronutrients**: Vitamin C, magnesium, and certain phytonutrients are limited on carnivores. Some rely on organ meats for variety, though not all choose to include them.

3. **Cholesterol & Heart Health**: Diets high in animal fats can raise LDL cholesterol in some individuals. Response varies, but monitoring with a healthcare professional is wise.

4. **Kidney & Liver Load**: High protein intake may be a concern for those with existing kidney disease. Medical oversight is strongly advised.

5. **Sustainability**: Many people use carnivore short-term as an elimination experiment, then transition to a more varied plan.

Since responses vary widely, it is best to approach these diets with professional guidance and ongoing monitoring. This helps ensure that any benefits are balanced with long-term safety and sustainability.

Choosing Between the Two

The decision between keto and carnivore often comes down to individual preference and tolerance.

- Those seeking structure, simplicity, and elimination of plant foods may experiment with carnivores.

- Those wanting metabolic benefits while keeping vegetables, nuts, and plant variety may choose keto.

Both approaches require attention to how the body responds. Blood work, digestion, energy, and overall wellbeing should guide adjustments. Importantly, anyone considering a major dietary shift should consult with a qualified healthcare provider, especially individuals who are pregnant, managing chronic illness, or taking medications that affect blood sugar or blood pressure.

Carnivore and keto share the possibility of ketosis, but they diverge in philosophy. Keto emphasizes flexibility within carb limits; carnivores emphasize restriction for simplicity or sensitivity reasons. Neither diet is universally superior. What matters is how sustainable, safe, and nourishing it feels for the individual.

Exploring these approaches with clinical guidance, self-awareness, and flexibility allows each person to find what supports their health best—whether that means the all-animal approach of carnivores, the mixed plant-and-animal approach of keto, or a middle ground between the two.

Who Should Not Follow the Carnivore Diet?

The carnivore diet is one of the most restrictive eating patterns, removing all plant foods and relying solely on animal products. For some, this simplicity feels appealing, but the limitations come with important risks. While a short-term elimination approach may be used by some under professional guidance, there are groups of people who should avoid this diet or approach it only with medical supervision.

Pregnant or Breastfeeding Women

Pregnancy and breastfeeding increase the body's nutrient demands. Vitamins such as folate, vitamin C, and a variety of plant-based antioxidants are especially important for fetal and infant development. Because the carnivore diet excludes fruits, vegetables, legumes, and whole grains, it can leave gaps in these critical nutrients.

Low intake of fiber may also worsen constipation, a common challenge during pregnancy. In breastfeeding mothers, reduced nutrient variety may affect milk quality. For these reasons, most health professionals recommend that pregnant or nursing women follow a balanced eating plan with a wide spectrum of food groups rather than an all-animal approach.

People with Kidney Disease

High intake of animal protein increases the workload on the kidneys. For individuals with healthy kidney function, this is usually not a concern. However, for those with chronic kidney disease (any stage) or reduced eGFR, a carnivore diet may place additional strain on already compromised kidneys.

Animal proteins can increase urea and other waste products that impaired kidneys struggle to filter, and they contribute to acid load, which may further challenge kidney function. Individuals with CKD should avoid restrictive high-protein diets like carnivore unless managed directly by a nephrologist or a qualified renal dietitian.

Those with Eating Disorders or a History of Disordered Eating

Restrictive diets can be triggering for people with current or past disordered eating patterns. The carnivore diet's rigid "all-or-nothing" rules may reinforce cycles of guilt, control, or obsession with food.

A healthy relationship with eating involves flexibility, variety, and social connection around meals. Eliminating entire food groups can heighten anxiety and reduce opportunities for balanced choices. For anyone with a history of anorexia, bulimia, binge eating disorder, or orthorexia, the carnivore diet is not advisable. Professional support from therapists and dietitians can help identify safer approaches that meet both physical and mental health needs.

Individuals Without Access to Nutrient-Dense Animal Foods

Not all animal products are equal in nutrient density. Grass-fed meats, organ meats, shellfish, and fatty fish provide a broader spectrum of vitamins, minerals, and omega-3 fats compared with highly processed meats. If a person relies only on budget cuts of red meat or processed products such as bacon and deli meats, nutrient gaps are more likely to appear.

In communities where fresh fish, eggs, or high-quality meats are limited or unaffordable, the carnivore diet becomes even more restrictive. Over time, this can raise the risk of deficiencies in vitamin C, magnesium, potassium, and other nutrients that plants typically supply. For individuals in these situations, the diet may be both impractical and nutritionally risky.

People Already in Good Health with No Symptoms to Resolve

The carnivore diet is often pursued as a short-term elimination strategy for digestive discomfort, autoimmune flares, or food sensitivities. However, for people who are generally healthy, with no ongoing symptoms or medical concerns, there is little reason to cut out entire food groups.

Adopting carnivores in such cases may remove valuable sources of fiber, antioxidants, and phytonutrients that support long-term health. A balanced diet that includes a variety of whole foods is typically more sustainable and provides broader protection against chronic disease.

The Role of Medical Supervision and Monitoring

Even in populations where the carnivore diet might be considered, medical oversight is essential. Blood tests to monitor cholesterol, kidney function, liver enzymes, vitamins, and minerals can help catch imbalances early. Healthcare professionals can also guide whether supplements or periodic reintroduction of plant foods are necessary to maintain balance.

Without this monitoring, risks such as nutrient deficiency, digestive issues, or metabolic strain may go unnoticed until they become more serious.

The carnivore diet is not appropriate for everyone. Pregnant or breastfeeding women, people with kidney disease, those with disordered eating histories, individuals without access to nutrient-dense animal products, and people already in good health with no reason to restrict should avoid or proceed with extreme caution.

For others, careful medical supervision and nutrient monitoring are non-negotiable. Any dietary pattern that removes entire food groups deserves thoughtful consideration, professional input, and an honest look at whether it can meet both short-term needs and long-term health goals.

The Benefits of the Carnivore Diet

The carnivore diet is one of the most restrictive eating patterns, centering meals exclusively on animal products. While its limits are obvious, many people who follow it share a surprising list of perceived benefits. These reports are not universal and have not been confirmed by long-term, large-scale clinical studies. Still, the recurring themes help explain why this diet has gained attention among people searching for simplicity, relief from certain food sensitivities, or a way to regulate appetite.

What follows is a closer look at the most commonly described outcomes. Each should be understood as anecdotal or observational—not guaranteed. Individual results vary widely, and anyone considering this diet should discuss it with a qualified healthcare professional before making major changes.

1. Reduced Cravings and Hunger

One of the first benefits people notice on carnivore is a sharp drop in food cravings. Meals made entirely of protein and fat tend to be highly satiating. Without the spikes and dips that can come from frequent carbohydrate intake, some report that they feel fuller for longer and no longer "graze" between meals.

For individuals who have struggled with cycles of overeating, this can feel liberating. The constant drive to snack or the pull toward sugary foods often lessens. Appetite seems steadier and easier to manage, which may explain why some people naturally cut down their total food intake without consciously restricting calories.

It is important to remember, however, that not everyone has the same appetite response. Some people thrive with steady fullness, while others miss the variety and satisfaction that different food textures and flavors bring.

2. Stable Blood Sugar and Fewer Energy Crashes

Another widely reported effect is more stable energy throughout the day. Because the carnivore diet eliminates nearly all dietary carbohydrates, blood sugar levels tend to remain more even. Without sharp rises after carb-heavy meals or dramatic drops a few hours later, many people say they feel steady energy without the afternoon "slump."

This steadiness is often linked to improved focus or mental clarity. People describe fewer energy crashes, less brain fog, and a smoother rhythm of alertness from morning to night.

That said, these experiences are not universal. Individuals with diabetes or those on medications affecting blood sugar should be especially cautious, as dietary shifts of this magnitude can alter medication needs. Medical supervision is essential in those cases.

3. Simplified Food Choices

Perhaps one of the most straightforward benefits is simplicity. For people overwhelmed by diets that require counting carbs, weighing food, or tracking macros, the carnivore approach cuts through the noise.

Decision fatigue—endlessly wondering "what should I eat?"—is greatly reduced. The rules are black and white: choose animal products. Some find this structure reassuring. Grocery shopping and meal prep can feel streamlined when the food list is short.

Simplicity also helps some people stick to the plan. Without hidden ingredients or constant label reading, compliance can feel more manageable compared with diets that require careful tracking.

The trade-off, however, is monotony. Over time, some miss the taste, color, and variety that vegetables, fruits, and grains bring to the table. For others, the simplicity outweighs the drawbacks.

4. May Support Weight Loss Through Appetite Regulation

Weight loss is a commonly discussed outcome on the carnivore diet. Because meals are filling and cravings often decline, many people naturally reduce how much they eat without counting calories. The diet is also nearly free of refined sugars and processed foods, which often drive overeating.

In addition, a carnivore plan is low in carbohydrates, which can lead to reduced water retention and initial weight shifts. Over time, some individuals continue to see fat loss, especially if appetite regulation keeps their calorie intake lower than before.

It is essential to stress that weight loss is not guaranteed. Success depends on many factors including metabolism, activity level, and underlying health conditions. Some individuals may lose weight quickly, while others may plateau or even gain if they eat large quantities of high-calorie foods such as cheese, cream, or fatty cuts of meat.

5. May Relieve Digestive Discomfort in Some People with IBS

Digestive relief is a common reason some individuals try the carnivore diet. For women with irritable bowel syndrome (IBS) or food sensitivities, removing fermentable plant fibers and naturally occurring compounds—like lectins or salicylates—may result in less bloating, cramping, or abdominal pain.

Because carnivore eliminates all plant foods, it also removes common digestive irritants in one step. This makes it functionally similar to a short-term elimination diet. Some women report more consistent digestion and fewer flare-ups when their food list is narrowed in this way.

Still, this response is not universal. While certain symptoms may ease, others may appear, such as changes in stool texture or frequency. These individual differences highlight that digestive comfort is highly personal—and that success with carnivore depends not just on what's removed, but also on how the body adapts in the absence of fiber and plant-based inputs.

The Role of Individual Variation

It is important to emphasize that these benefits are not experienced by everyone. Some feel energized, leaner, and less symptomatic, while others feel fatigued, restricted, or uncomfortable. Outcomes depend heavily on genetics, metabolism, gut health, and personal preferences.

Even among those who report benefits, many do not stay on the diet indefinitely. Some use carnivore for a short-term reset or as an elimination trial, then transition to a more varied plan that reintroduces tolerated foods.

Putting Benefits in Context

The carnivore diet is best understood not as a guaranteed path to health but as an approach that may work for a select group of people under the right circumstances. The simplicity, appetite regulation, and potential digestive relief explain its appeal. Still, the absence of plant-based nutrients raises questions about long-term balance and safety.

For individuals curious about trying carnivore, a cautious mindset is wise:

- Work with a qualified healthcare professional to monitor health markers.
- Pay attention to energy, digestion, and mood, and make adjustments if negative symptoms appear.
- Be open to transitioning to a more balanced approach if long-term sustainability is difficult.

The carnivore diet is unconventional, restrictive, and highly debated. Yet, for some, it provides real-life benefits such as reduced cravings, steadier energy, simplified choices, potential weight loss, and digestive relief. These reported outcomes highlight why it has found a loyal following, even without widespread scientific endorsement.

Everybody responds differently. What feels like freedom and relief for one person may feel monotonous or limiting for another. Understanding these nuances ensures that the conversation around carnivore remains realistic and respectful of individual experience.

More Benefits for Women on the Carnivore Diet

When women consider dietary changes, the focus often goes beyond weight or appetite. Energy, mood, skin health, and hormone balance play equally important roles. Advocates of the carnivore diet often highlight unique benefits that appear especially meaningful for women.

While these outcomes are reported frequently, they remain anecdotal or observational. They vary widely between individuals, and nutritional adequacy is critical to prevent unwanted hormone disruptions or deficiencies.

1. Skin Appearance and Reduced Sugar Intake

One of the most frequently mentioned anecdotal changes among women who try a carnivore-style plan is a shift in skin appearance. Some report clearer or calmer skin, which may be related to the removal of refined sugars and ultra-processed foods—both of which are excluded on the diet.

High sugar intake has been linked in research to higher insulin levels, shifts in androgen activity, and increased sebum production, factors that can contribute to acne in certain individuals. However, skin health is influenced by many variables including genetics, hormones, stress, sleep, and skincare routines. While dietary change may play a role for some, evidence remains limited, and not everyone notices a difference.

It is worth noting that not all skin concerns are diet-related. Stress, sleep, hormones, and skincare routines are also important. Still, many women see reduced inflammation or puffiness when sugar and processed foods are minimized, and carnivore guarantees their removal.

2. Fewer PMS Symptoms and More Stable Moods

Another commonly reported benefit is a shift in premenstrual symptoms. Limited evidence and personal accounts indicate some women may experience fewer mood swings, less bloating, or reduced cramps. The reasons are not entirely clear. Some speculate that stable blood sugar levels, higher intake of fats for hormone production, and the removal of plant-based irritants may play a role.

Mood stability is another area often highlighted. Without the rapid energy spikes and dips that can come from carbohydrate fluctuations, women sometimes feel calmer, more even, and less prone to irritability. Whether related to ketosis, macronutrient balance, or simply eating fewer processed foods, the perceived benefit is notable.

Again, not all women experience this change. Hormonal cycles are complex, and many factors influence PMS. But for some, carnivore creates an environment where symptoms feel less disruptive.

Low-Carb Eating and PCOS: What Some Women Report

Polycystic ovary syndrome (PCOS) is closely associated with insulin resistance. Research on moderate or low-carbohydrate eating patterns suggests they may help support healthier insulin and androgen dynamics in some women. A number of women with PCOS have shared anecdotal reports of improved cycle regularity, fewer cravings, or easier weight management when carbohydrate intake is reduced.

Because the carnivore diet eliminates virtually all carbohydrates, some individuals experimenting with it also describe changes in cycle patterns or energy. However, these accounts remain observational, and strict zero-carb or all-animal approaches have not been directly studied in PCOS. Most published research still includes some plant foods.

Each woman's hormonal profile is unique, and outcomes vary widely. Medical guidance is essential before attempting major dietary changes, particularly with a restrictive plan like carnivore. For those who choose to try it, carnivore is best viewed as a short-term elimination experiment under professional supervision, with close attention to nutrient adequacy, blood work, and symptom tracking.

1. **High-Fat Intake and Hormone Synthesis**

   Fats play a central role in hormone production, particularly estrogen and progesterone. Many women find reassurance in the fact that carnivore naturally provides high dietary fat. Animal-based fats, cholesterol, and fat-soluble vitamins act as building blocks for steroid hormones.

   For women who have struggled with very low-fat diets in the past, the higher intake on carnivore may feel stabilizing. Some describe fewer mood fluctuations or more consistent menstrual cycles when their diet contains abundant fat sources such as fatty cuts of beef, lamb, or salmon.

Still, balance matters. Excess saturated fat without the balance of plant nutrients can bring concerns for cardiovascular health. A moderate, individualized approach under professional supervision is advised.

2. Mental Clarity and Emotional Regulation

Cognitive and emotional changes are also reported. Women sometimes describe sharper concentration, fewer "brain fog" episodes, and greater emotional steadiness. This is often linked to steady ketone production, which can provide a reliable fuel source for the brain.

Emotional regulation may also improve simply because energy highs and lows are minimized. For women who feel reactive or fatigued on high-carb diets, the carnivore approach can feel like a smoother ride.

As with other benefits, not all experiences are positive. Some women feel depleted without the variety of plant-based nutrients. This reinforces the importance of ongoing monitoring and individualization.

Nutritional Adequacy and Hormonal Health

The potential benefits of carnivore must be balanced with awareness of nutritional adequacy. While animal foods provide many essential nutrients, certain vitamins, minerals, and phytonutrients are less available without plant foods. For women, this raises special considerations:

- **Folate**: Essential for reproductive health; typically abundant in leafy greens but limited on carnivore.

- **Vitamin C**: Plays a role in collagen synthesis and immune support; scarce without plant sources.

- **Magnesium and Potassium**: Important for mood regulation and muscle function; more easily obtained from plant foods.

If these nutrients are insufficient, hormone stability may suffer rather than improve. That is why many women who explore carnivore treat it as a temporary elimination tool, later reintroducing foods to round out nutrient intake.

The Individual Factor

The most important lesson from women's experiences with carnivore is variability. Some thrive, feeling more stable, clearer, and lighter. Others feel deprived, fatigued, or hormonally off balance. Personal context—age, metabolic health, activity level, and stress—shapes how the body responds.

For those curious, the safest approach is gradual experimentation under guidance. Tracking cycle health, mood, and energy over time provides clues about whether the diet is supporting or straining the body.

The carnivore diet remains controversial, but for some women, it appears to bring meaningful benefits. Skin improvements, steadier moods, reduced PMS, potential PCOS support, stronger hormonal foundations from dietary fat, and mental clarity are among the most reported outcomes.

Still, these benefits are not guaranteed and should not overshadow the importance of nutritional adequacy. Without attention to nutrients like folate, vitamin C, and magnesium, long-term health may be compromised.

For women, the carnivore diet may offer a short-term reset or an elimination framework to identify food sensitivities. But lasting wellness usually depends on balance, flexibility, and individualized care. With professional guidance and close self-observation, women can decide whether this path enhances their health—or whether a more varied approach better supports their body's needs.

Potential Risks and Nutrient Gaps

The carnivore diet can feel deceptively simple: eat meat, fish, eggs, and animal fats, and eliminate everything else. This clarity appeals to many women who are exhausted by tracking calories, weighing foods, or navigating long "do and don't" lists. Yet like any restrictive diet, carnivore carries risks. While some women report increased energy, reduced bloating, or improved skin, others encounter challenges ranging from mild digestive changes to significant nutrient gaps. Understanding these risks is crucial before committing fully to this eating style.

The goal here is not to discourage women from exploring carnivore, but to provide a balanced view so choices are made with awareness. No single diet suits everyone, and what feels empowering for one person may be problematic for another. By reviewing potential pitfalls — and outlining ways to monitor, adapt, or seek professional guidance — women can approach carnivore more safely and sustainably.

Micronutrient Gaps

Animal foods are nutrient-dense, offering protein, iron, zinc, vitamin B12, vitamin A, and essential fatty acids. Still, a carnivore diet excludes many plant-based sources of vitamins and minerals. This creates the possibility of gaps, particularly in:

- **Vitamin C**: Traditionally sourced from fruits and vegetables, vitamin C plays a role in collagen production, wound healing, and immune support. Small amounts exist in raw organ meats and fish roe, but intake may not reach levels considered sufficient by most health authorities. Women may not notice a deficiency immediately, but longer-term absence can increase risk of fatigue, gum irritation, or impaired recovery from minor injuries.

- **Folate** – Essential for DNA synthesis, red blood cell health, and reproductive function. Folate is found in leafy greens, legumes, and fortified grains. While liver does provide folate, relying on it alone carries limitations, especially if consumed inconsistently or in small amounts.

- **Magnesium** – This mineral supports hundreds of enzymatic processes, including nerve function, muscle contraction, and blood pressure regulation. Most dietary magnesium comes from nuts, seeds, and leafy greens, which are absent from carnivore. Animal foods contain small amounts, but deficiencies can develop over time, sometimes manifesting as muscle cramps, poor sleep, or irritability.

- **Potassium** – A key electrolyte for fluid balance, nerve impulses, and heart function. Potassium is plentiful in fruits, vegetables, and beans, but relatively low in most meats. Symptoms of deficiency can include fatigue, muscle weakness, or heart rhythm changes.

These potential gaps underscore why carnivore should not be undertaken without supervision. Women may benefit from periodic blood tests to check nutrient status. If shortfalls are identified, strategies such as consuming organ meats more consistently or carefully selected supplements under professional guidance may help.

Fiber Elimination

On a carnivore diet, all dietary fiber is removed—along with the plant foods that provide it. While some individuals welcome the shift, especially those with fiber sensitivity, others may find the change challenging.

Fiber supports bowel regularity, stool bulk, and microbial fermentation in the colon. Without it, digestion often shifts. Some women notice smaller, less frequent stools, or increased effort during elimination. In contrast, others find that removing fiber reduces gas, bloating, or urgency—especially if their gut previously reacted poorly to fermentable plant fibers.

Whether digestion improves or worsens depends on multiple factors, including hydration, electrolyte intake, and fat consumption. When fiber is removed, water balance in the intestines changes. Supporting hydration with salt, broth, and dietary fat can help. Some women use magnesium under clinical guidance to maintain bowel comfort.

The key is not to assume that fiber removal is automatically helpful or harmful—it's to observe your body's specific response and make adjustments based on how digestion feels day to day.

Cholesterol and Heart Health

A carnivore diet typically relies on fatty cuts of meat, eggs, butter, and tallow. While these foods provide energy and fat-soluble vitamins, they are also high in saturated fat and cholesterol. The clinical impact varies:

- **For some women:** Blood markers remain stable or even improve, particularly triglycerides and HDL cholesterol, which can benefit metabolic health.

- **For others:** LDL cholesterol rises sharply, potentially increasing cardiovascular risk depending on genetics and underlying health.

This variability makes monitoring essential. Regular lipid panels, ideally before and during carnivore, help track how the body responds. Women with a family history of heart disease, high cholesterol, or metabolic conditions should be especially cautious. Balance can be achieved by incorporating a variety of animal foods, not relying solely on red meat, and including fish rich in omega-3 fatty acids like salmon or sardines.

It is important to remember that cardiovascular risk is influenced by many factors beyond diet: genetics, activity level, stress, and sleep all play roles. Carnivore may fit within a healthy lifestyle for some women, but without oversight, it carries real risks for others.

Hormonal Disruption

Hormones are closely influenced by nutrition, energy intake, and body composition. While some women report improvements on the carnivore diet — such as fewer PMS complaints or more predictable cycles — restrictive eating patterns can also create new challenges if not approached carefully.

- **Caloric intake:** Because food choices are limited, some women unintentionally undereat. Persistently low energy intake may contribute to irregular cycles, reduced fertility signals, or worsening fatigue. Tracking overall calories and ensuring adequate protein and fat can help reduce this risk.

- **Carbohydrate scarcity:** Very low carbohydrate intake may influence thyroid function and reproductive hormones in some individuals. While many women adapt well, others may notice changes such as irregular cycles, hair shedding, or mood fluctuations. These shifts can signal the need to adjust intake or consider a less restrictive approach.

- **Protein–fat balance:** Adequate dietary fat is essential for hormone production. Focusing too heavily on lean meats while neglecting fattier cuts, seafood, or egg yolks may limit the building blocks needed for estrogen, progesterone, and other steroid hormones.

Hormonal responses vary greatly between women and across life stages. Women of reproductive age should pay attention to menstrual patterns, while those approaching or in menopause may require different nutritional strategies.

Tracking changes in cycles, mood, and energy — and discussing them with a qualified healthcare provider — offers the clearest picture of whether the carnivore approach is supporting or straining hormonal health.

Navigating These Risks Safely

Awareness of risks does not mean abandoning carnivore entirely. Instead, it invites a thoughtful, flexible approach. Here are strategies that may help mitigate pitfalls:

- **Medical oversight:** Partner with a doctor or dietitian familiar with low-carb and elimination diets. Request baseline and follow-up labs to check nutrient levels, cholesterol, and thyroid markers.

- **Organ meats in rotation:** Liver, heart, kidney, and marrow provide diverse nutrients missing from muscle meat. However, avoid excessive liver intake to prevent vitamin A overload.

- **Electrolyte balance:** Salt food generously, drink adequate fluids, and consider magnesium or potassium support if advised by a clinician.

- **Diversity within limits:** Rotate between beef, lamb, pork, poultry, and seafood to avoid relying on one source. Fish rich in omega-3s can balance high saturated fat intake from ruminant meats.

- **Monitor energy and cycles:** Track physical, emotional, and hormonal changes. If fatigue, irregular cycles, or mood instability appear, adjust food intake or consider transitioning to a less restrictive plan.

The Role of Supplements

While carnivore emphasizes whole animal foods, supplementation may still have a place, especially for women. Common considerations include:

- **Magnesium** for sleep and muscle relaxation.

- **Vitamin C** for collagen support and immune health.

- **Electrolytes** to maintain hydration and nerve function.

Not every woman will need these, but supplement use should always be tailored, guided by blood work and professional advice. Self-experimentation without context can create more problems than it solves.

The carnivore diet can feel liberating in its simplicity, but simplicity does not equal safety. Women considering this approach must weigh the benefits against potential risks. Micronutrient shortfalls, digestive changes, cholesterol shifts, and hormonal disruptions are real possibilities. These risks do not automatically disqualify the diet, but they highlight the importance of awareness, balance, and medical oversight.

Every woman's physiology, history, and goals are unique. A diet that energizes one woman may deplete another. By approaching carnivore with caution, monitoring responses closely, and making adjustments as needed, women can explore this path without compromising their long-term health.

14-Day Guide to Stick to the Carnivore Diet Plan

Starting the carnivore diet can feel both exciting and intimidating. Unlike most eating patterns, it strips food choices down to animal-based sources only—meat, fish, eggs, and sometimes dairy—removing every plant-based food. This simplicity can feel freeing but also requires an adjustment period as your body adapts to new fuel sources.

The following 14-day guide is designed to help women transition with structure and realistic expectations. It outlines common adaptation symptoms, practical strategies to manage them, and sample meals to simplify planning. With patience, self-awareness, and medical guidance, the first two weeks can lay the foundation for a smoother experience.

Adaptation Period

The first one to two weeks on the carnivore diet are often the most challenging. This phase, sometimes called the "adaptation period," reflects the body's shift from carbohydrate-based fuel toward primarily fat and ketones.

While this metabolic transition is natural, it can trigger uncomfortable symptoms. Knowing what to expect can help you approach the process with patience and reassurance.

Common Symptoms

- **Headaches and Brain Fog:** As carbohydrate intake plummets, glycogen stores in the liver and muscles become depleted. This shift can temporarily alter hydration and electrolyte balance, leading to headaches or a cloudy, unfocused feeling known as "brain fog."

- **Fatigue and Irritability:** The body is used to glucose as its primary energy source. When that is suddenly removed, energy production feels unstable. Many women report feeling unusually tired, less motivated, or more irritable during this stage.

- **Sleep Disruption:** Falling asleep or staying asleep can be harder during the early days of carb restriction. Some women experience restlessness or vivid dreams. Sleep usually improves as the body adjusts to burning fat more efficiently.

- **Cravings for Carbohydrates or Sugar:** These are among the most difficult hurdles. Your body, accustomed to a steady stream of glucose, sends signals urging you to reach for bread, fruit, or sweets. This is not a sign of failure but rather a natural response to change.

- **Digestive Changes:** Fiber intake drops to nearly zero on carnivore, which can create noticeable shifts in bowel habits. Some women develop constipation, while others experience loose stools or diarrhea. This occurs as the digestive system adjusts to the absence of plant fibers and the increased presence of dietary fats.

Why These Symptoms Happen

The root of these changes is metabolic adaptation. As glycogen stores empty, water and electrolytes are lost with them. Meanwhile, the digestive tract and gut microbiome are adjusting to a new environment. These symptoms are not usually dangerous but can feel discouraging. They tend to improve by the end of the second week as the body becomes more efficient at using fat for fuel and restoring balance.

Key takeaway: For many women, early adaptation symptoms improve within a couple of weeks. With proper support and realistic expectations, energy and cravings often stabilize. If fatigue, digestive issues, or other concerns persist or worsen, it's important to reassess the plan with your clinician.

Coping with These Changes

Transition symptoms can be discouraging, but there are practical ways to ease the discomfort and help the body adapt more smoothly.

1. **Hydrate Generously**

   Water needs often increase during the first weeks because glycogen depletion causes more water loss. Aim for steady hydration throughout the day rather than large amounts at once. Warm beverages like broth can be especially soothing and hydrating.

2. **Add Salt and Electrolytes**

   Electrolyte shifts are a key cause of headaches, fatigue, and irritability during adaptation. Many people feel better with higher sodium intake in the first weeks, as glycogen and water losses increase salt needs. Exact requirements vary, so discuss an appropriate range with your healthcare professional. Magnesium or potassium support should only be used under clinical guidance, especially if you take blood pressure or diuretic medications.

3. **Eat More Animal Fat**

   Low energy is often a sign of not eating enough fat. Lean meats alone may leave you feeling weak. Choose ribeye, salmon, or add tallow, butter, or ghee to meals.

Adequate fat helps fuel ketone production and promotes satiety.

4. Avoid Fasting at First

While intermittent fasting is popular in low-carb communities, combining fasting with the early adaptation period can worsen fatigue and cravings. In the first two weeks, eat when hungry—even if that means three or four meals per day. Once your energy stabilizes, fasting can be revisited.

5. Rest and Lower Exercise Intensity

Overtraining during adaptation can leave you drained. Strength workouts may feel harder, and endurance may suffer temporarily. Gentle movement, stretching, or walking are ideal during this period. Save higher-intensity training for after your body has adjusted.

6. Practice Patience and Self-Awareness

This stage is temporary, but the symptoms can feel discouraging. Remind yourself that these reactions are part of your body learning to run on a new fuel source. Tracking your energy, digestion, and mood in a simple journal can help you see progress and stay motivated.

Managing hydration, electrolytes, fat intake, and rest can dramatically reduce adaptation discomfort. With patience and gentle self-care, most women find symptoms fade by the second week.

Easing into the Carnivore Diet

Transitioning to an all-animal food plan can feel overwhelming if attempted overnight. Many people find success by gradually approaching carnivore gradually. A stepwise method allows the body to adapt, reduces potential discomfort, and gives beginners time to evaluate how they feel at each stage. The following framework offers a flexible path rather than a rigid prescription.

Step 1: Remove Processed Foods and Added Sugar

The first step is clearing out processed foods and added sugars. This includes sodas, packaged snacks, pastries, candy, and heavily refined convenience meals. These foods tend to create cycles of cravings, unstable blood sugar, and excess hunger. By removing them, you begin to reset taste buds and appetite signals.

During this stage, there's no need to restrict all carbohydrates. The focus is on replacing highly processed foods with more whole, nutrient-dense options. Instead of sweetened cereal, start the day with eggs. Replace fast-food lunches with grilled chicken or salmon. Have fruit instead of candy if you still want something sweet.

This stage can last one to two weeks, or longer if needed. The goal is to lay the foundation for steadier energy and less reliance on quick sugar hits. Many people notice fewer mid-afternoon crashes just by cutting soda and desserts. Once cravings for processed food begin to fade, you'll feel more prepared to make further adjustments.

Step 2: Focus on Whole Animal-Based Proteins

After cutting processed foods, the next step is to make animal-based proteins the anchor of every meal. This doesn't yet require eliminating vegetables or grains, but it shifts your plate toward the foods that will become central later.

Aim for each meal to include a solid portion of meat, fish, or eggs. Breakfast might be scrambled eggs with a side of bacon, lunch could be grilled chicken with a salad, and dinner might feature a steak with roasted vegetables. By building around protein, you naturally reduce reliance on breads, pastas, and filler foods.

This stage isn't about strict elimination but about shifting priorities. It helps regulate appetite by giving the body more of the macronutrient that provides satiety. Women especially may find this stabilizing, since adequate protein supports both muscle preservation and hormone production.

Over a week or two, you may notice that the desire for starchy sides or snacks diminishes as protein intake rises. You'll also begin to recognize which foods keep you full and which ones leave you sluggish—insights that will help when moving toward low-carb eating.

Step 3: Move Into Low-Carb or Keto

Once protein is central, the next phase is shifting into a low-carb or ketogenic style of eating for one to two weeks. This means reducing daily carb intake significantly, typically by cutting out bread, pasta, rice, and most fruits, while keeping non-starchy vegetables like spinach, zucchini, and cauliflower.

The purpose of this step is to help the body adapt to using fat as fuel. When carbs drop, the body begins producing ketones from fat. This metabolic switch can feel uncomfortable at first—commonly described as "keto flu"—and may involve fatigue, irritability, or headaches. Allowing one to two weeks in this stage gives time for adaptation.

Electrolyte balance becomes especially important during this stage. Many people feel better with higher sodium intake as carbohydrate restriction leads to water and salt losses. Exact needs vary, so it is best to discuss an appropriate range with a healthcare professional. Magnesium or potassium support should only be considered under clinical guidance, especially if you take medications such as diuretics or those affecting blood pressure. Staying well-hydrated and prioritizing sleep can also ease the transition.

By the end of this stage, many notice more stable energy and fewer cravings. With the body already fat-adapted, the transition to carnivore feels smoother and less abrupt.

Step 4: Gradually Reduce Plant Foods

After the body has adapted to low-carb eating, the next step is to gradually reduce plant foods. This stage highlights whether certain vegetables, nuts, or fruits trigger digestive discomfort, bloating, or skin issues. It also prepares digestion for the eventual removal of plant fiber.

Start by eliminating starchier vegetables and fruits such as potatoes, carrots, bananas, and apples. Keep lighter, low-carb options such as leafy greens or cucumbers for now. Over time, continue reducing until only a small selection of tolerated vegetables remains. Nuts, seeds, and plant-based oils can also be phased out during this stage.

This is often the most eye-opening step, as it provides a clear sense of how different foods affect the body. Some people notice reduced bloating or less abdominal discomfort, while others miss the variety and fiber. Because digestion changes when fiber is reduced, it allows time for the body to adapt.

This step can last as long as needed. Some pause here and never go further, finding that a very-low-carb diet without most plants works best for them. Others continue on to full carnivore once they feel ready.

Step 5: Transition to Full Carnivore

The final step is adopting a fully animal-based diet, where meals consist only of meat, fish, eggs, and, in some versions, dairy. By this stage, the body is generally fat-adapted and less reliant on carbohydrates, which makes the transition less abrupt than starting from a standard diet.

Meals can stay straightforward: eggs and bacon for breakfast, grilled salmon for lunch, and a ribeye steak for dinner. Pay attention to hydration and electrolytes, since mineral balance shifts when plant foods are excluded. Some people add organ meats for extra nutrients, while others stick to basic cuts of meat.

Many begin with a short trial—commonly 30 days—to observe changes in digestion, appetite, energy, or mood. Some extend the plan longer, while others use it briefly as an elimination reset before reintroducing selected foods.

Throughout this stage, track your own signals. Feeling steady and satisfied may indicate the approach is working, but fatigue, discomfort, or signs of deficiency suggest adjustments are needed. For some, that means modifying the plan; for others, returning to a low-carb or ketogenic pattern works better.

Not everyone needs to reach full carnivore to experience benefits. The gradual, stepwise path offers natural checkpoints to pause, reflect, and decide whether continuing makes sense. With professional guidance and a flexible mindset, you can settle on the level of carbohydrate restriction that supports your health most effectively.

Sample 14-Day Guide

This two-week sample provides a simple structure for easing into carnivore eating. Meals focus on meat, eggs, and broth without sauces, sides, or complicated preparation. Portions can be adjusted to individual appetite.

Week 1

Day 1

Breakfast: Scrambled eggs with ground beef

Lunch: Grilled chicken thighs

Dinner: Ribeye steak

Day 2

Breakfast: Fried eggs

Lunch: Ground beef patties

Dinner: Salmon fillet

Day 3

Breakfast: Omelet with ground beef

Lunch: Chicken thighs

Dinner: Sirloin steak

Day 4

Breakfast: Hard-boiled eggs

Lunch: Salmon

Dinner: Ground beef patties

Day 5

Breakfast: Scrambled eggs

Lunch: Chicken thighs

Dinner: Ribeye steak

Day 6

Breakfast: Fried eggs with liver

Lunch: Ground beef patties

Dinner: Salmon fillet

Day 7

Breakfast: Omelet with chicken thigh pieces

Lunch: Beef steak

Dinner: Bone broth with soft-boiled eggs

Week 2

Day 8

Breakfast: Scrambled eggs

Lunch: Ground beef patties

Dinner: Salmon

Day 9

Breakfast: Fried eggs with liver

Lunch: Chicken thighs

Dinner: Ribeye steak

Day 10

Breakfast: Omelet with beef

Lunch: Salmon fillet

Dinner: Ground beef patties

Day 11

Breakfast: Hard-boiled eggs

Lunch: Chicken thighs

Dinner: Beef steak

Day 12

Breakfast: Scrambled eggs with liver

Lunch: Ground beef patties

Dinner: Salmon

Day 13

Breakfast: Fried eggs

Lunch: Chicken thighs

Dinner: Ribeye steak

Day 14

Breakfast: Omelet with ground beef

Lunch: Salmon fillet

Dinner: Bone broth with eggs

Grocery Shopping Tips

Shopping for carnivore eating is straightforward, but choosing wisely improves both nutrient intake and budget efficiency.

- **Prioritize fatty cuts:** Ribeye, pork belly, lamb shoulder, duck legs, and salmon provide energy-dense fat and flavor.

- **Include organ meats:** Liver, kidney, and heart supply vitamins and minerals not always abundant in muscle meat.

- **Buy in bulk:** Large packages of ground beef, roasts, or whole chickens are often more affordable. Freeze in portions for later use.

- **Use bones:** Bones and marrow are inexpensive yet nutrient-rich. They make excellent broth, which also supports hydration.

- **Look for minimally processed meats:** Choose cuts without added sugar, fillers, or seed oils. Sausages and deli meats should be checked carefully for additives.

- **Optional grass-fed:** Grass-fed or pasture-raised meats are encouraged if accessible, but they are not mandatory. Nutritional adequacy can still be achieved with conventional cuts.

A weekly grocery trip focused on fatty meats, eggs, fish, and broth ingredients covers nearly all essentials for the first 14 days.

Foods Included in the Carnivore Diet Plan

The carnivore diet permits a wide range of animal-based foods. Commonly included:

- **Red meats:** Beef, lamb, pork, venison, bison

- **Poultry:** Chicken, turkey, duck

- **Fish and shellfish:** Salmon, sardines, shrimp, crab, mussels

- **Organ meats:** Liver, kidney, heart, brain, tongue

- **Eggs:** Whole eggs, prepared any style

- **Animal fats:** Bone marrow, tallow, suet, duck fat

- **Bone broth** for hydration and minerals

- **Optional dairy:** Butter, heavy cream, ghee, and hard cheeses if tolerated

Some women prefer a "strict" approach with only meat, salt, and water. Others include butter, cream, or cheese for flexibility. The choice depends on individual goals, tolerance, and health considerations.

Foods to Avoid

Carnivore eating is defined by exclusion. Foods to avoid include:

- **Fruits and vegetables:** Typically all types, including leafy greens and berries, are excluded.

- **Legumes and grains:** Beans, lentils, rice, oats, and wheat are generally removed.

- **Sugar and sweets:** Candy, soda, baked goods, and other added-sugar foods are avoided.

- **Processed snacks:** Chips, crackers, and granola bars are not usually included.

- **Seed oils:** Many people on carnivore choose to limit oils such as soybean, canola, corn, sunflower, and safflower. If used, selecting minimally processed versions and monitoring personal tolerance can be a balanced approach.

- **Optional eliminations:** Coffee and tea are debated; stricter practitioners exclude them to remain fully animal-based.

This exclusion is not about declaring plant foods "bad." Instead, it functions as an elimination tool to identify potential irritants and create a controlled environment. Some women later reintroduce select foods to test tolerance.

Sample 7-Day Carnivore Diet Meal Plan

The following plan offers a straightforward structure to help you visualize what a week of carnivore eating can look like. Meals are kept simple, repetitive, and easy to prepare. Portions are not specified—eat until comfortably satisfied. The goal is to rotate between beef, pork, poultry, lamb, and fish while varying lean and fatty cuts for balance. Bone broth, tallow, and butter can be added for extra hydration and energy.

Day 1

- **Breakfast:** Bacon and fried eggs cooked in tallow

- **Lunch:** Ribeye steak with salt

- **Dinner:** Grilled salmon with a cup of bone broth

Day 2

- **Breakfast:** Scrambled eggs with butter (or ghee if dairy-free)

- **Lunch:** Pork belly slices, pan-seared until crispy

- **Dinner:** Roast lamb chops with rendered fat drizzled over top

Day 3

- **Breakfast:** Beef liver sautéed in butter with two eggs

- **Lunch:** Ground beef patties (80/20 blend) with optional melted cheese

- **Dinner:** Roast chicken thighs with skin, served with warm broth made from chicken bones

Day 4

- **Breakfast:** Hard-boiled eggs with crispy pork cracklings

- **Lunch:** Slow-cooked beef brisket, sliced and served with broth

- **Dinner:** Pan-seared duck breast with rendered fat

Day 5

- **Breakfast:** Omelet made with eggs and heavy cream (optional dairy)

- **Lunch:** Grilled shrimp or scallops cooked in butter

- **Dinner:** Ribeye steak with marrow bones on the side

Day 6

- **Breakfast:** Bacon and poached eggs

- **Lunch:** Lamb shoulder roast, slow-cooked until tender

- **Dinner:** Grilled salmon or sardines, finished with melted tallow or butter

Day 7

- **Breakfast:** Fried eggs with leftover brisket slices

- **Lunch:** Pork ribs, oven-baked and lightly salted

- **Dinner:** Ground beef meatballs (optionally blended with heart or liver) simmered in bone broth

Tips for Success

- **Batch cooking helps:** Preparing brisket, ribs, or lamb shoulder in larger portions provides multiple meals.

- **Vary fat levels:** Alternate fattier cuts (ribeye, pork belly, lamb shoulder) with leaner options (chicken breast, shrimp) to balance satiety and energy.

- **Use broth daily:** Bone broth can be a helpful source of hydration and sodium. Its mineral content varies widely depending on preparation, so it should be seen as a supportive beverage rather than a primary mineral source..

- **Rotate proteins:** Mixing beef, poultry, pork, lamb, and fish ensures a broader range of nutrients.

This 7-day sample is not intended to be prescriptive but to show how simple, repeatable meals can build structure. Women often find that sticking to a few staple foods during the first week reduces decision fatigue and makes adaptation easier.

Long-Term Sustainability and Alternatives

The carnivore diet is one of the most restrictive eating approaches, cutting away entire categories of foods that most people have grown up eating daily. For women drawn to its simplicity, symptom relief, or clear rules, it can feel like a lifeline. Yet the very features that make carnivore appealing in the short term can become barriers in the long term. Social isolation, nutrient gaps, cravings, or plateaued progress are common realities after the first months of enthusiasm fade.

This chapter explores what "sustainability" truly means, why rigid approaches can create new problems, and what alternatives women can consider when carnivore no longer feels supportive.

Why Sustainability Matters

Sustainable nutrition is not just about sticking with a diet for life; it's about living in a way that supports health, enjoyment, and adaptability. Women face unique challenges across life stages — from menstrual cycles and fertility to menopause and bone health. A diet that feels doable in one phase may not meet the demands of another.

Carnivore offers a reset for many women by stripping away triggers, irritants, and decision fatigue. However, sustainability requires a plan beyond the elimination phase. Without that plan, what begins as empowering can shift into rigidity, nutrient imbalance, or social stress.

The Plateau Effect

A common story among women who try carnivore is dramatic initial improvement — clearer skin, steady energy, or quick weight loss — followed by a plateau. Over time, the body adapts, symptoms may resurface, or new issues emerge. Constipation, hair shedding, or menstrual irregularities can appear months into carnivore, even if the first weeks felt effortless.

Plateaus do not necessarily mean failure; they often signal that it is time to reassess. Health is dynamic, and nutrition must be flexible enough to evolve alongside it.

Cyclical Carnivore

One approach to sustainability is a **cyclical carnivore model**, in which strict animal-only eating is practiced for a set period, followed by the reintroduction of select plant foods.

1. **Seasonal eating:** Some women add berries in the summer, herbs in small amounts, or cooked tubers occasionally. This mirrors ancestral patterns of food availability while giving the body periodic exposure to phytonutrients and fiber.

2. **Symptom testing:** Reintroductions can also serve as experiments. For example, a woman who eliminated all plants to calm digestion may test small amounts of zucchini, cucumber, or avocado to see if symptoms return.

This cyclical pattern can preserve many benefits of carnivore — reduced processed food, steady appetite control, simplified decision-making — while softening its rigidity.

Keto or Low-Carb Alternatives

For women who thrive on low-carb living but feel constrained by strict carnivore, transitioning to **keto or low-carb** eating can be a practical alternative.

- **Variety with control:** Keto expands the food palette to include leafy greens, low-sugar fruits, nuts, seeds, and dairy. This makes it easier to meet micronutrient needs while still keeping blood sugar and insulin stable.

- **Flexibility for life stages:** Women entering perimenopause or managing thyroid concerns may find that slightly higher carbohydrate intake supports hormone balance.

- **Balance with social life:** Eating out, sharing meals with family, or enjoying occasional treats becomes less stressful in a keto or low-carb framework compared to strict carnivore.

This shift does not negate the benefits gained from carnivore; instead, it builds upon them by layering in flexibility and variety.

Targeted Elimination Diets

Another sustainable path is a **targeted elimination diet**, where the goal is not to avoid all plant foods but to identify and exclude specific triggers.

- **Common triggers:** Gluten, dairy, soy, and certain legumes are frequent culprits in digestive distress, skin flare-ups, or fatigue.

- **Structured reintroduction:** Women can begin with a broad elimination (such as Whole30, AIP, or modified paleo) and then reintroduce foods one at a time to test tolerance.

- **Personalization:** This approach acknowledges that food reactions are individual. While one woman may thrive without dairy, another may tolerate it perfectly but struggle with grains.

Targeted elimination protects against unnecessary restriction while still honoring the principle of food-as-data: eat, observe, and adjust.

Psychological and Social Factors

Sustainability is not just biological; it is emotional and social. Many women describe feeling socially isolated on carnivore, especially during holidays, family gatherings, or travel. Constantly explaining food rules can be tiring, and over time, the rigidity may increase stress rather than reduce it.

A sustainable approach acknowledges the importance of shared meals and social connection. Allowing occasional flexibility — whether that means coffee with friends, enjoying a piece of fruit, or sharing a holiday dish — may support long-term adherence better than absolute rigidity.

Signs It May Be Time to Transition

Every woman's body offers feedback. Signs that strict carnivore may no longer be serving include:

- Persistent constipation or digestive discomfort.

- Menstrual irregularities or worsening PMS.

- Unexplained fatigue, hair thinning, or mood instability.

- Rising cholesterol or concerning lab results.

- Strong cravings, binge episodes, or growing resentment of food rules.

These signals do not always mean carnivore is "wrong," but they indicate the need for evaluation. Adjustments could be as small as adding more fat, diversifying protein sources, or reintroducing specific plant foods.

Periodic Reassessment

Long-term sustainability requires regular check-ins. A practical rhythm is to reassess every three to six months by asking:

- Are my original symptoms still improved?

- Have new problems emerged?

- How is my energy, mood, and cycle health?

- Are my labs within a healthy range?

- Does this way of eating still feel empowering, or does it feel like a burden?

These reflections help prevent dogma from taking over. A diet is a tool, not an identity. If carnivore no longer fits, it is not a failure — it is simply information.

Building Flexibility Into the Future

The most sustainable approach often blends lessons from carnivore with the broader principles of balanced nutrition. Women may discover that certain foods truly cause problems and are best avoided, while others can be enjoyed without consequence. The long-term goal is not perfection but resilience: a way of eating that adapts to life's seasons, stresses, and joys.

By experimenting with cyclical carnivore, transitioning into keto or low-carb, or adopting targeted elimination diets, women can preserve the clarity and benefits of carnivore while avoiding its pitfalls.

The carnivore diet offers a dramatic reset for some women, but it is not always designed for lifelong use. Over time, rigidity can lead to nutrient gaps, social strain, or hormonal challenges. Sustainability comes from flexibility, balance, and the courage to evolve.

Women are encouraged to honor both the benefits they have experienced and the signals their bodies provide when it is time for change. Cyclical approaches, keto, low-carb, or targeted elimination diets can extend the lessons of carnivore into a broader, more balanced lifestyle.

Ultimately, the best diet is one that nourishes both body and spirit — today, and for the years ahead.

Sample Recipes

Cooking on the carnivore diet is refreshingly simple. With just a handful of ingredients—meat, eggs, animal fat, and salt—you can prepare meals that are nourishing, satisfying, and surprisingly varied. The focus is not on elaborate seasonings or side dishes, but on highlighting the natural flavors of high-quality animal foods.

This recipe collection offers straightforward ways to prepare beef, pork, poultry, lamb, and seafood, with options ranging from quick skillet meals to slow-cooked roasts. Each recipe uses minimal ingredients, stays true to the carnivore framework, and can be adjusted for either strict or flexible versions of the diet. The goal is to make everyday cooking effortless, while still providing the variety needed to stay consistent with this way of eating.

Simple Beef Burgers

Servings: 2–3 burgers

Prep Time: 5 minutes

Cook Time: 8–10 minutes

Ingredients:

- 1 lb ground beef (80/20 preferred for fat content)
- Salt to taste
- *Optional:* 2 oz minced liver for nutrient boost

Instructions:

1. Combine ground beef (and liver if using) in a mixing bowl. Shape into patties about ½–¾ inch thick.
2. Heat a skillet or grill pan over medium-high heat.
3. Cook patties for 3–4 minutes per side for medium, adjusting for preferred doneness.
4. Sprinkle it with salt and serve hot.

Strict carnivore note: *Serve plain. Avoid condiments or seasonings beyond salt.*

Roasted Brisket

Servings: 6–8

Prep Time: 10 minutes

Cook Time: 4–5 hours

Ingredients:

- 3–4 lb beef brisket
- Salt to taste
- *Optional:* 2 tbsp beef tallow for basting

Instructions:

1. Preheat the oven to 300°F (150°C).
2. Rub brisket generously with salt.
3. Place brisket in a roasting pan. Add tallow if desired for moisture.
4. Cover tightly with foil and roast for 4–5 hours, until the meat is fork-tender.
5. Let rest 15 minutes before slicing.

Strict carnivore note: *Avoid using marinades. Tallow or broth are safe moisture boosters.*

Liver with Butter

<u>**Servings**</u>: 2

<u>**Prep Time**</u>: 5 minutes

<u>**Cook Time**</u>: 5 minutes

Ingredients:

- 8 oz beef or chicken liver, sliced thin
- 2 tbsp butter or ghee (*omit for strict carnivore*)
- Salt

Instructions:

1. Heat butter or ghee in a skillet over medium heat.
2. Add liver slices. Cook 2–3 minutes per side, until browned but still tender inside.
3. Season lightly with salt and serve immediately.

Strict carnivore note: *Cook liver in beef tallow instead of butter for a dairy-free option.*

Safety note: *Liver is very high in vitamin A. To avoid excess intake, most clinicians recommend limiting beef liver to about **1–2 servings per week**. Pregnant individuals should discuss liver intake with their healthcare professional before including it regularly.*

Grilled Shrimp

<u>**Servings**</u>: 2

<u>**Prep Time**</u>: 5 minutes

<u>**Cook Time**</u>: 6 minutes

Ingredients:

- 1 lb shrimp, peeled and deveined
- 1 tbsp butter or beef tallow
- Salt

Instructions:

1. Preheat grill or skillet to medium-high heat.
2. Toss shrimp with melted butter or tallow and sprinkle with salt.
3. Cook 2–3 minutes per side until pink and firm.
4. Serve hot.

Strict carnivore note: *Use tallow instead of butter if avoiding dairy.*

Lamb Chops

<u>**Servings**</u>: 2

<u>**Prep Time**</u>: 5 minutes

<u>**Cook Time**</u>: 8–10 minutes

Ingredients:

- 4 lamb chops
- 1 tbsp tallow or ghee
- Salt

Instructions:

1. Heat skillet over medium-high heat and add tallow.
2. Season lamb chops with salt.
3. Sear 3–4 minutes per side for medium-rare, adjusting for doneness preference.
4. Rest for 5 minutes before serving.

Strict carnivore note: *Serve simply, without herbs or marinades.*

Bacon-Wrapped Salmon

Servings: 2

Prep Time: 5 minutes

Cook Time: 18–20 minutes

Ingredients:

- 2 salmon fillets
- 4 slices bacon
- Salt to taste

Instructions:

1. Preheat the oven to 375°F (190°C).
2. Wrap each salmon fillet with 2 slices of bacon, overlapping slightly to secure.
3. Place wrapped fillets on a parchment-lined baking sheet.
4. Bake for 18–20 minutes, until the bacon is crisp and salmon flakes easily.
5. Season with salt and serve immediately.

Strict carnivore note: *Ensure bacon is free of sugar or additives.*

Bone Broth

Servings: 6–8 cups

Prep Time: 10 minutes

Cook Time: 12–24 hours

Ingredients:

- 2 lb beef or chicken bones (marrow, knuckles, or joint bones recommended)
- *Optional:* 2 tbsp vinegar (helps extract minerals)
- Salt to taste

Instructions:

1. Place bones in a large stock pot. Cover completely with water.
2. Add vinegar if using, then bring to a gentle simmer.
3. Simmer uncovered for 12–24 hours, skimming off foam or impurities as needed.
4. Strain liquid into jars or a container. Season with salt before serving.
5. Store in the refrigerator for up to 5 days or freeze for longer.

Strict carnivore note: *Skip vinegar if aiming for a purist approach.*

Shredded Chicken in Broth

Servings: 4

Prep Time: 10 minutes

Cook Time: 1–2 hours

Ingredients:

- 1 whole chicken or 4 chicken thighs
- 8 cups water
- Salt to taste

Instructions:

1. Place chicken in a large pot. Cover fully with water.
2. Bring to a simmer and cook gently for 1–2 hours, until chicken is cooked through.
3. Remove chicken from the pot. Shred meat into bite-sized pieces.
4. Return shredded meat to the broth.
5. Season with salt and serve warm.

Strict carnivore note: *Stick to skin, meat, and broth only. Avoid vegetables or spices.*

Steak with Tallow

<u>Servings</u>: 1–2

<u>Prep Time</u>: 5 minutes

<u>Cook Time</u>: 8–10 minutes

Ingredients:

- 1 ribeye or sirloin steak
- 2 tbsp beef tallow
- Salt to taste

Instructions:

1. Heat a heavy skillet or cast-iron pan over medium-high heat. Add tallow and let it shimmer.
2. Pat steak dry, season with salt.
3. Sear 3–4 minutes per side for medium-rare (adjust for thickness).
4. Transfer steak to a cutting board and rest for 5 minutes.
5. Slice and serve hot, spooning rendered tallow over top if desired.

Strict carnivore note: *Use only salt; avoid marinades or pepper.*

Duck Breast with Rendered Fat

<u>**Servings**</u>: 2

<u>**Prep Time**</u>: 5 minutes

<u>**Cook Time**</u>: 10–12 minutes

Ingredients:

- 2 duck breasts
- Salt to taste

Instructions:

1. Pat duck breasts dry. Score skin in a crosshatch pattern, being careful not to cut into meat.
2. Place breasts skin-side down in a cold skillet. Turn heat to medium.
3. Cook for 6–8 minutes, allowing fat to render and skin to become crisp.
4. Flip and cook an additional 3–4 minutes until desired doneness.
5. Rest for 5 minutes before slicing. Spoon rendered fat over meat when serving.=

Strict carnivore note: *Serve plain—duck fat itself provides rich flavor.*

Pork Belly Crisps

<u>Servings</u>: 2–3

<u>Prep Time</u>: 5 minutes

<u>Cook Time</u>: 25–30 minutes

Ingredients:

- 1 lb pork belly, sliced into strips
- Salt to taste

Instructions:

1. Preheat the oven to 400°F (200°C).
2. Arrange pork belly slices on a parchment-lined baking sheet.
3. Season lightly with salt.
4. Roast for 25–30 minutes, flipping halfway, until golden and crisp.
5. Drain excess fat and serve hot.

Strict carnivore note: *Avoid commercial bacon with additives—stick to plain pork belly.*

Sardines with Butter

Servings: 1–2

Prep Time: 2 minutes

Cook Time: 3 minutes

Ingredients:

- 1 can sardines (in water or olive oil, drained)
- 1 tbsp butter (or tallow for strict version)

Instructions:

1. Warm a skillet over medium heat.
2. Add butter or tallow, then sardines.
3. Heat 2–3 minutes until warm.
4. Serve immediately.

Strict carnivore note: *Choose sardines packed in water, not oil, to avoid plant-based ingredients.*

Roasted Bone Marrow

<u>**Servings**</u>: 2–3

<u>**Prep Time**</u>: 5 minutes

<u>**Cook Time**</u>: 15–20 minutes

Ingredients:

- 4 marrow bones, cut lengthwise
- Salt

Instructions:

1. Preheat the oven to 425°F (220°C).
2. Place bones marrow-side up on a baking tray.
3. Roast 15–20 minutes until marrow bubbles.
4. Sprinkle with salt and scoop out with a spoon.

Strict carnivore note: *Eat as-is or spread marrow over steak for added fat.*

Shrimp & Egg Scramble

Servings: 2

Prep Time: 5 minutes

Cook Time: 5 minutes

Ingredients:

- 6 eggs, beaten
- ½ lb shrimp, chopped
- 2 tbsp butter or tallow
- Salt

Instructions:

1. Heat butter in a skillet over medium heat.
2. Add shrimp and cook until pink, about 2 minutes.
3. Pour in beaten eggs and scramble until just set.
4. Season with salt and serve hot.

Strict carnivore note: *Skip butter and use tallow for dairy-free strictness.*

Slow-Cooked Lamb Shoulder

Servings: 4–6

Prep Time: 10 minutes

Cook Time: 8 hours (slow cooker)

Ingredients:

- 3–4 lb lamb shoulder
- Salt

Instructions:

1. Rub lamb with salt.
2. Place in a slow cooker and cook on low for 8 hours, or until tender.
3. Shred meat and serve with its juices.

Strict carnivore note: *Cook without added herbs or vegetables.*

Beef Heart Steaks

Servings: 2–3

Prep Time: 10 minutes

Cook Time: 6 minutes

Ingredients:

- 1 lb beef heart, trimmed and sliced into steaks
- 1 tbsp beef tallow
- Salt

Instructions:

1. Heat tallow in a skillet over medium-high heat.
2. Season heart slices with salt.
3. Sear 2–3 minutes per side until browned but tender.
4. Serve immediately.

Strict carnivore note: *Simple salt only—avoid marinades.*

Chicken Thighs with Crispy Skin

<u>**Servings**</u>: 2–3

<u>**Prep Time**</u>: 5 minutes

<u>**Cook Time**</u>: 40–45 minutes

Ingredients:

- 4 chicken thighs, skin-on
- Salt

Instructions:

1. Preheat the oven to 375°F (190°C).
2. Pat thighs dry and season with salt.
3. Roast 40–45 minutes until the skin is crisp and juices run clear.
4. Rest 5 minutes before serving.

Strict carnivore note: *Serve plain, without sauces or seasoning blends.*

Ground Beef Meatballs in Broth

Servings: 3–4

Prep Time: 10 minutes

Cook Time: 12 minutes

Ingredients:

- 1 lb ground beef (80/20)
- 4 cups bone broth
- Salt

Instructions:

1. Form ground beef into small meatballs and season lightly with salt.
2. Bring bone broth to a simmer in a saucepan.
3. Drop meatballs into broth and cook for 10–12 minutes until done.
4. Serve meatballs in broth for a simple, hearty meal.

Strict carnivore note: *No breadcrumbs or binders—just beef.*

Crispy Chicken Skin "Chips"

Servings: 2

Prep Time: 5 minutes

Cook Time: 15–20 minutes

Ingredients:

- Chicken skin pieces (saved from thighs or breasts)
- Salt

Instructions:

1. Preheat the oven to 400°F (200°C).
2. Lay chicken skin flat on a parchment-lined sheet.
3. Sprinkle it with salt.
4. Bake for 15–20 minutes until crisp.
5. Cool slightly before serving for maximum crunch.

Strict carnivore note: *Store extras in the fridge and re-crisp in the oven if needed.*

Pan-Seared Scallops

Servings: 2

Prep Time: 5 minutes

Cook Time: 4 minutes

Ingredients:

- 8 scallops, patted dry
- 1 tbsp butter or tallow
- Salt

Instructions:

1. Heat fat in a skillet over high heat until it shimmers.
2. Place scallops in pan and sear 1–2 minutes per side until golden.
3. Sprinkle it with salt and serve immediately.

Strict carnivore note: *Use tallow instead of butter for strict carnivore.*

Beef Tongue Slices

<u>**Servings**</u>: 4

<u>**Prep Time**</u>: 10 minutes

<u>**Cook Time**</u>: 2–3 hours (simmering)

Ingredients:

- 1 beef tongue
- Salt

Instructions:

1. Place tongue in a large pot, cover with water, and simmer for 2–3 hours until tender.
2. Remove and peel off the thick outer skin.
3. Slice the tongue thinly.
4. Pan-sear slices briefly in their own fat before serving.

Strict carnivore note: *Eat warm or cold—tongue is nutrient-dense and versatile.*

Duck Fat Omelet

Servings: 1–2

Prep Time: 5 minutes

Cook Time: 4 minutes

Ingredients:

- 3 eggs
- 1 tbsp duck fat
- Salt

Instructions:

1. Heat duck fat in a skillet over medium heat.
2. Beat eggs, season with salt, and pour into skillet.
3. Cook until just set, folding once.
4. Serve immediately.

Strict carnivore note: *Skip cream or cheese—eggs and fat alone keep it carnivore.*

Making the Change for Better Health

Choosing to adopt a restrictive plan such as the carnivore diet is never just about food. For many women, it represents a search for stability — in energy, mood, digestion, or weight — after years of trial and error with different eating patterns. The process is not simply nutritional; it also involves mindset, motivation, and self-awareness.

This section offers encouragement for those considering the carnivore diet, while also providing balanced insights into other approaches. The goal is to empower women to make choices that feel sustainable, safe, and personally meaningful.

Why Women Turn Toward Change

Many women come to the carnivore diet after years of frustration with chronic fatigue, bloating, stubborn weight gain, or cyclical mood changes. These issues often persist despite "clean eating" or traditional diet strategies. For some, the simplicity of a meat-only plan feels refreshing. There are no complicated recipes, no need to log every calorie, and fewer decisions to make throughout the day.

The structured nature of the plan can feel motivating, giving meals a predictable rhythm. Even if followed only briefly, this framework helps women notice patterns in digestion, energy, and mood that inform later food choices.

Potential Benefits Women Report

Women who experiment with carnivore frequently describe improvements that extend beyond the scale. While outcomes are not universal, several patterns emerge in personal accounts and survey data:

- **Clarity of thought**: Many women describe less "brain fog," possibly due to stable blood sugar and reduced intake of refined carbohydrates.

- **Digestive calm**: Some report that cutting plant fibers or processed foods helps ease bloating or IBS-like symptoms.

- **Mood balance**: Low sugar intake and more stable energy may contribute to fewer mood swings, particularly around the menstrual cycle.

- **Reduced cravings**: Eating mostly protein and fat appears to increase satiety, helping some women step off the cycle of constant snacking.

- **Energy stability**: Without large carbohydrate swings, energy may feel steadier across the day.

These reports are valuable for understanding motivation, but it's important to emphasize they are anecdotal. Not every woman experiences these changes, and some encounter new challenges, such as constipation, low energy during exercise, or menstrual cycle disruptions.

Reducing Processed Foods

Regardless of whether someone adopts carnivore fully, one undeniable advantage is the **removal of processed food and sugar**. Modern diets are often loaded with refined carbohydrates, industrial oils, and packaged snacks that provide calories but little nourishment.

When these foods are cut out, women often experience:

- **Steadier blood sugar**: Limiting refined carbs reduces post-meal crashes.

- **Less inflammation**: Highly processed foods are linked to chronic low-grade inflammation, which plays a role in fatigue and metabolic health.

- **Better appetite control**: Processed foods are engineered to be hyper-palatable, making it hard to stop at a reasonable portion. Removing them can quiet cravings.

- **Improved skin**: For some women, less sugar and fewer additives correlate with fewer breakouts or flare-ups of skin conditions like acne.

In this way, the carnivore diet works as an **extreme reset**. By eliminating nearly all potential irritants, it forces the diet back to basics. For some, this allows the body to recalibrate.

Listening to Your Body

The structured nature of carnivore can feel reassuring, with clear guidelines that remove much of the guesswork. Yet this same rigidity can backfire if it overrides the body's natural signals.

For long-term health, it is crucial to maintain awareness of how your body responds. Questions to ask include:

- *Am I feeling nourished and energized, or run down?*

- *Has my digestion improved, or become more sluggish?*

- *Is my menstrual cycle regular and predictable, or showing disruptions?*

- *Am I eating enough overall, or sliding into restriction because of limited options?*

Tracking these signals can help determine whether the diet is serving you or causing unintended stress. If energy is low, if cycles are changing, or if mood feels flat, that is information — not failure. Listening to these cues and adjusting accordingly is part of taking ownership of your health.

The Role of Flexibility

Some women thrive on carnivore for months or years, while others view it as a short-term elimination tool. It is perfectly valid to treat it as a temporary experiment rather than a permanent lifestyle.

A useful mindset is to see carnivore as a laboratory. By stripping the diet to its simplest form, it becomes easier to notice how the body reacts when foods are added back in. For example:

- If dairy is reintroduced and bloating returns, that's valuable insight.

- If leafy greens are added without discomfort, that may signal a tolerance worth keeping.

- If small amounts of berries support energy and digestion without negative effects, they may belong in the long-term plan.

This approach transforms carnivore from a restrictive rulebook into a **tool for self-discovery**.

Other Approaches Worth Considering

Carnivore is one path, but it is not the only way to simplify eating or explore food sensitivities. Some women may find success with more flexible approaches, such as:

- **Elimination diets**: Removing common triggers like gluten, dairy, soy, and added sugar, then reintroducing systematically.

- **Carb cycling**: Incorporating low-carb eating most days but adding higher-carb meals once or twice per week to support hormones and energy.

- **Whole-food keto**: A gentler version of carnivore that includes low-carb vegetables, nuts, and berries.

- **Paleo or primal**: Emphasizing whole, unprocessed foods while allowing fruits, vegetables, and natural fats.

Each of these approaches offers structure without the extreme restriction of carnivore. Women who are hesitant about removing all plant foods may find these alternatives more sustainable.

Personalization Is the Key

No single diet works for every woman. Genetics, medical history, activity level, and life stage all shape dietary needs. For example:

- Women approaching menopause may need more protein to protect bone and muscle mass.

- Women with thyroid conditions may not tolerate very low-carb eating for extended periods.

- Active women or athletes may require carbohydrate flexibility to fuel performance.

- Women with histories of eating disorders may find extreme restriction triggering.

This is why medical supervision is essential. Blood tests, nutrient monitoring, and regular check-ins with a provider ensure that the body is supported rather than depleted.

Motivation Beyond the Plate

Food is only part of the story. Sustainable change also depends on mindset and environment. A few strategies that help women stay motivated include:

- **Reframing success**: Rather than focusing only on the scale, pay attention to energy, mood, sleep quality, and digestion.

- **Building routines**: Meal prepping, grocery shopping lists, and structured eating times reduce decision fatigue.

- **Community support**: Sharing experiences with others who are experimenting can make the process less isolating.

- **Celebrating progress**: Small wins, such as fewer cravings or steadier energy, deserve recognition.

Motivation deepens when women view dietary change not as punishment, but as an experiment in self-care.

The Reality Check

While carnivore can feel transformative for some, it is not a magic solution. Risks include nutrient deficiencies (vitamin C, folate, magnesium), potential increases in LDL cholesterol for certain individuals, and long-term questions about gut microbiome diversity.

Acknowledging these risks does not invalidate the benefits women report — it simply ensures decisions are made with clear eyes. A responsible approach balances short-term gains with long-term health.

Encouragement for the Journey

Dietary change is rarely a straight line. Some days will feel easy and empowering, while others may feel restrictive or frustrating. The most important message is that **there is no one-size-fits-all answer**.

For women seeking relief from fatigue, bloating, or unstable mood, the carnivore diet may provide insights or temporary improvement. For others, a less restrictive plan may be more appropriate. The key is to remain curious, compassionate with yourself, and willing to adjust along the way.

In the end, making the change for better health is about more than following rules. It's about regaining trust in your body, understanding your unique needs, and building an approach that feels nourishing, not punishing. Whether that involves strict carnivores, a hybrid model, or another path altogether, the power lies in personalization.

Conclusion

Adopting the carnivore diet as a woman is less about rigid rules and more about gaining insight into how your body responds to food. Streamlining meals to animal foods alone creates a structured way to test for sensitivities and sometimes brings short-term improvements in appetite balance, skin clarity, or digestion.

Yet those benefits come with real considerations. Nutrient gaps in vitamin C, folate, magnesium, and potassium are possible. Hormonal health may be affected if energy intake is too low or fat intake is unbalanced. Long-term sustainability depends on flexibility, not strict adherence alone.

As you move forward, listen closely to your energy, cycles, digestion, and mood. These signals are feedback, not failures. If you feel empowered, stable, and clear-headed, then the approach may be serving you. If you notice fatigue, irregular cycles, or digestive discomfort, consider modifications such as rotating different cuts of meat, adding organ meats, or experimenting with cyclical or keto alternatives. Always involve a healthcare professional when making these decisions. Regular check-ins and lab work protect against hidden deficiencies or metabolic shifts.

Use the carnivore diet as a learning tool, not a permanent label. Many women discover that a short trial provides clarity about which foods feel supportive and which trigger discomfort. From there, you can reintroduce selected foods strategically, design a cyclical pattern, or transition to a broader low-carb approach. This flexibility protects against social isolation, nutrient depletion, and the mental strain of long-term rigidity.

Ultimately, your health journey is personal. The carnivore diet can serve as one experiment among many, but it is not the final destination for most. What matters most is sustainability—finding a way of eating that nourishes you physically, emotionally, and socially. Approach this path with curiosity, patience, and compassion for yourself. By treating the process as an exploration rather than a prescription, you give yourself permission to adapt, evolve, and create a plan that supports you at every stage of life.

FAQs

What's the simplest way to start?

Begin with a 1–2 week clean-up: remove sugar and ultra-processed foods, build each meal around meat, eggs, or fish, and add broth. If you feel steady, step down to low-carb/keto for 1–2 weeks, then trial full carnivore.

How much should I eat?

Aim for adequate protein first (rough guide: ~1.2–1.6 g/kg body weight/day, or follow your clinician's advice). Let fat provide the rest of your energy—choose fattier cuts if you feel low energy or hungry between meals.

Do I need extra salt or electrolytes?

Many people feel better with added sodium during adaptation. Salt food to taste, sip broth, and consider magnesium or potassium only with clinician guidance—especially if you take blood pressure or diuretic medications.

How do I prevent constipation without plant fiber?

Hydrate, salt adequately, and include enough dietary fat (very lean menus can slow stools). Bone broth may help; some use clinician-approved magnesium. If symptoms persist, reassess the plan with your provider.

Is dairy okay for carnivores?

Some people include dairy on a carnivore-style plan, while stricter versions exclude it. If you choose to experiment, start with simpler options such as butter, ghee, hard cheeses, or plain heavy cream. Monitor carefully for any changes in digestion, skin, or congestion, and adjust as needed. Because dairy tolerance varies widely, it's best to make decisions in consultation with a healthcare professional—especially if you have lactose intolerance, allergies, or hormonal concerns.

What labs should I monitor—and how often?

Discuss a baseline and follow-up panel with your clinician (e.g., lipid profile/ApoB, fasting glucose/A1c, CMP, CBC, ferritin/iron studies, B12/folate, vitamin D, thyroid panel, and electrolytes). Recheck after 8–12 weeks and adjust your plan accordingly.

Will this affect my menstrual cycle or hormones?

Possibly. Undereating or going very low-carb can disrupt cycles for some; prioritize enough total calories and fat, track symptoms, and involve your healthcare professional if cycles change or PMS worsens.

References and Helpful Links

Baker, S. (2019). *The Carnivore Diet*. Victory Belt Publishing.

O'Hearn, A., & Peterson, P. (2020). Nutritional considerations of zero-carbohydrate diets. *Journal of Evolutionary Health*, 5(2), 1–15.

Smith, R., Johnson, L., & Lee, K. (2021). Low-carbohydrate diets and female hormone regulation: A review. *Nutrition Reviews*, 79(11), 1201–1215.

Peterson, C. M., & Nadeau, K. J. (2020). Dietary carbohydrate restriction and insulin resistance. *Frontiers in Endocrinology*, 11, 350.

Gibson, P. R., & Shepherd, S. J. (2010). Evidence-based dietary management of functional gastrointestinal symptoms: The FODMAP approach. *Journal of Gastroenterology and Hepatology*, 25(2), 252–258.

Astrup, A., & Geiker, N. R. W. (2019). Saturated fat and cardiovascular disease: Is a revision of the recommendations warranted? *Current Opinion in Clinical Nutrition & Metabolic Care*, 22(6), 451–457.

Westman, E. C., Volek, J. S., & Phinney, S. D. (2020). Low-carbohydrate diets for managing obesity and metabolic disease: Evidence review. *Nutrition & Metabolism*, 17, 92.

www.ingramcontent.com/pod-product-compliance
Lightning Source LLC
Chambersburg PA
CBHW031251250726
48655CB00005B/2172